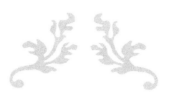

# The Type 2 Diabetic Cookbook

A Detailed Beginners Guide To Diabetic Diet To Kickstart Your Healthy Living With Type 2 Diabetes By Cracking The Code, And Reversing Diabetes Without Drugs

Isabella Miller

the author is not engaging in the rendering of legal, financial, medical or professional advice. The content within this book has been derived from various sources. Please consult a licensed professional before attempting any techniques outlined in this book.

By reading this document, the reader agrees that under no circumstances is the author responsible for any losses, direct or indirect, which are incurred as a result of the use of information contained within this document, including, but not limited to, errors, omissions, or inaccuracies.

# Table of Contents

# Breakfast and Brunch

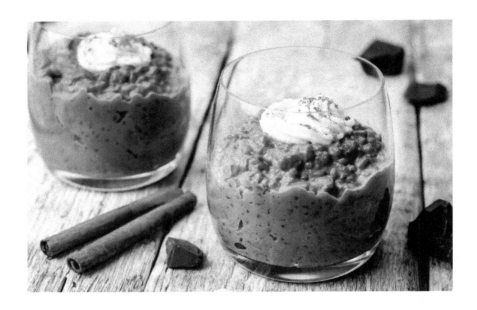

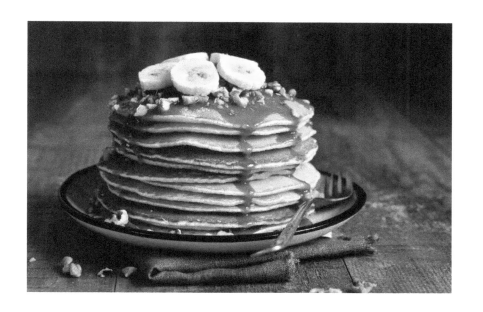

**1. Breakfast Beans**
**Preparation Time:** 15 minutes
**Cooking Time:** 10 minutes
**Servings:** 2
**Total budget**: 5

## Ingredients
- 1 lb. baked beans
- 1 lb. mixed lean meat, chopped
- 1 cup eggs, scrambled
- 1 tbsp. mixed herbs
- 2 stalks scallions

## Directions
Mix all the ingredients in your Instant Pot, cook on Stew for 10 minutes. Release the pressure naturally.

## Nutrition
**Calories:** 300 kcal    **Total Fat:** 7 g    **Protein:** 42 g

## 2. Sausage Breakfast Casserole
**Preparation Time:** 15 minutes
**Cooking Time:** 10 minutes
**Servings:** 2
**Total budget**: 9

### Ingredients
- 1 lb. sausage, cooked and chopped
- 1 lb. bell pepper and onions, chopped
- 1 cup low sodium broth
- 1 tbsp. mixed herbs
- 1 tbsp. Soy sauce

### Directions
Mix all the ingredients in your Instant Pot, cook on Stew for 10 minutes. Release the pressure naturally.

### Nutrition
**Calories:** 360 kcal   **Total Fat:** 24 g   **Protein:** 35 g

### 3. Coconut Pancakes
**Preparation Time:** 25 minutes
**Cooking Time:** 25 minutes
**Servings:** 2
**Total budget**: 4$

### Ingredients
- 1 cup coconut milk, unsweetened
- ¼ tsp. sea salt
- ½ cup coconut flour
- ½ tsp. baking soda
- 4 eggs, lightly beaten
- ½ tsp. vanilla extract, pure
- 3 tbsps. olive oil

### Directions
Whisk all your ingredients and then melt a tbsp. oil into a skillet using medium heat. Add your batter in and cook for two to three minutes per side. Use up all your batter and serve warm.

### Nutrition
**Calories:** 340 kcal   **Total Fat:** 29 g   **Protein:** 10 g

## 4. Blueberry Matcha Smoothie
**Preparation Time:** 5 minutes
**Cooking Time:** 5 minutes
**Servings:** 2
**Total budget**: 7$

### Ingredients
- 2 cups blueberries, frozen
- 2 cups almond milk
- 1 banana
- 2 tbsps. protein powder, optional
- ¼ tsp. ground cinnamon
- 1 tbsp. chia seeds
- 1 tbsp. Matcha powder
- ¼ tsp. ground ginger
- A pinch sea salt

### Directions
Blend everything until smooth.

### Nutrition
**Calories:** 208 kcal   **Total Fat:** 5.7 g   **Protein:** 8.7 g

## 5. Pumpkin Pie Smoothie
**Preparation Time:** 5 minutes
**Cooking Time:** 5 minutes
**Servings:** 2
**Total budget**: 6$

### Ingredients
- 1 banana
- ½ cup pumpkin, canned & unsweetened
- 2-3 ice cubes
- 1 cup almond milk
- 2 tbsps. almond butter, heaping
- 1 tsp. ground nutmeg
- 1 tsp. ground cinnamon
- 1 tsp. vanilla extract pure

### Directions
Blend everything until smooth.

### Nutrition
**Calories:** 235 kcal     **Total Fat:** 11 g     **Carbs:** 27.8 g
**Protein:** 5.6 g

## 6. Leek & Spinach Frittata
**Preparation Time:** 25 minutes
**Cooking Time:** 25 minutes
**Servings:** 2
**Total budget:** 10

## Ingredients
- 2 leeks, chopped fine
- 2 tbsps. avocado oil
- 8 eggs
- ½ tsp. garlic powder
- ½ tsp. basil, dried
- 1 cup baby spinach, fresh & packed
- 1 cup Cremini mushrooms, sliced
- Sea salt & black pepper to taste

## Directions
Heat oven to 400°F and then get out an ovenproof skillet. Place it over medium-high heat, sautéing your leeks in your avocado oil until soft. It should take roughly five minutes. Get out a bowl, and whisk the eggs with your garlic, basil, and salt. Add them to the skillet with your leeks, cooking for five minutes. You will need to stir frequently. Stir in your mushrooms and spinach, seasoning with pepper. Place skillet in the oven, baking for ten minutes. Serve warm.

## Nutrition
**Calories:** 276 kcal     **Total Fat:** 17 g     **Carbs:** 15 g
**Protein:** 19 g

**7. Fig Smoothie**
**Preparation Time:** 5 minutes
**Cooking Time:** 5 minutes
**Servings:** 2
**Total budget**: 5$

## Ingredients
- 7 figs, halved (fresh or frozen)
- 1 banana
- 1 cup whole milk yogurt, plain
- 1 cup almond milk
- 1 tsp. flaxseed, ground
- 1 tbsp. almond butter
- 1 tsp. honey, raw
- 3–4 ice cubes

## Directions
Blend everything until it will be smooth and serve immediately.

## Nutrition
**Calories:** 362 kcal    **Total Fat:** 12 g    **Protein:** 9 g

# Lunch Vegetable Recipes

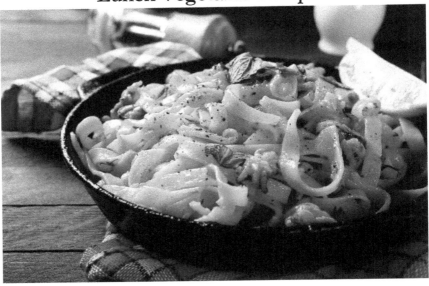

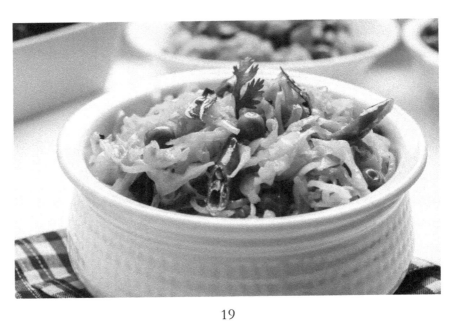

**1. White Bean and Bacon Soup**
**Preparation Time:** 15 min
**Cooking Time:** 2 hrs
**Servings:** 2
**Total budget**: 10$
**Ingredients**

- 3 cups chicken bouillon
- 2 cups beans
- 4 slices medium-cut bacon
- 2 carrots
- 2 celery, stalks
- ¾ cup onion
- 1 clove garlic, chopped
- ¼ tsp. pepper
- ½ tsp. salt
- 1 bay leaf

**Directions**

Soak the beans before cooking in water for 8 hours. Place washed beans into the Instant Pot, then fry chopped bacon in a skillet over medium heat until it becomes crisp. Take bacon from skillet and mill it into small pieces. Add chopped carrot, onion, celery, and garlic in skillet; cook until vegetables are tender. Shift cooked mixture and bacon into the Instant Pot. Add bouillon, salt, pepper, and bay leaf. Cook until beans are tender.

**Nutrition**
**Calories:** 80 kcal   **Total Fat:** 4 g   **Protein:** 2 g

## 2. Braised White Beans with Baby Kale

**Preparation Time:** 20 min
**Cooking Time:** 1h 20 min
**Servings:** 2
**Total budget**: 15$
**Ingredients**

- 1 (5-oz.) baby kale
- 1 (15-oz.) can bean with no salt
- 1 (15-oz.) can tomatoes, diced
- 1 tbsp. extra virgin olive oil
- ½ cup onion, chopped
- 1 clove garlic
- ½ tsp. oregano, dried
- 2 cups low-sodium vegetable broth

## Directions

Heat virgin olive oil over medium heat in a large pan. Add onion, oregano, and minced garlic, cook 10 minutes (stirring often). Add vegetable broth and bring to a boil. Cook 6 to 8 minutes. Append drained and rinsed beans and tomatoes; reduce heat to medium-low and cook 40 minutes, stirring occasionally. Combine with kale; cook, constantly stirring, until kale wilts. I love cooking this dish for my family.

## Nutrition

**Calories:** 60 kcal    **Total Fat:** 1 g    **Protein:** 6 g

## 3. Quick Kidney Bean Soup with Cheese

**Preparation Time:** 10 min

**Cooking Time:** 10 min

**Servings:** 2

**Total budget**: 10$

**Ingredients**

- 1 (15-oz.) can kidney beans, no-salt-added
- ¼ cup cheese, shredded, reduced-fat
- ⅓ cup Picante sauce
- ⅓ cup green onions
- 1 tsp. paprika, smoked
- ⅔ cup water
- 2 tsps. extra virgin olive oil

**Directions**

Mix drained and rinsed beans, picante sauce, smoked paprika, and water in a small saucepan; bring to a boil. Reduce heat, simmer for 5 minutes. Remove from heat and stir in oil. Top soup evenly with 2 tbsps. cheese and chopped green onions. A good way to gain a flat belly or to keep your current shape!

**Nutrition**

**Calories:** 56 kcal   **Total Fat:** 1 g   **Protein:** 4 g

## 4. Herbed Potato and Green Bean

**Preparation Time:** 10 min
**Cooking Time:** 13 min
**Servings:** 2
**Total budget:** 10$

### Ingredients

- ½ lb. potatoes
- ½ lb. green beans
- ½ tsp. Rosemary, dried
- 1 tbsp. extra virgin olive oil
- 1 tsp. lemon juice
- ⅓ tsp. salt
- 1 tsp. pepper

### Directions

Arrange potatoes and green beans in a steamer basket over boiling water. Cover and steam for 10 to 13 minutes. Carry vegetables to a bowl; mix with olive oil, lemon juice, crushed rosemary, salt, and pepper. An easy recipe that will surprise everyone!

### Nutrition

**Calories:** 66 kcal    **Total Fat:** 0 g    **Protein:** 3 g

# Lunch Meat Recipes

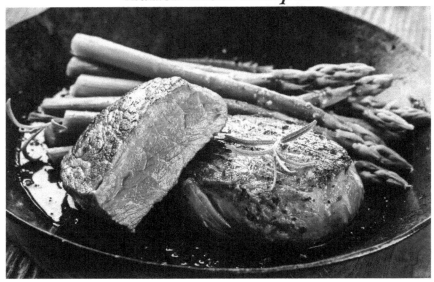

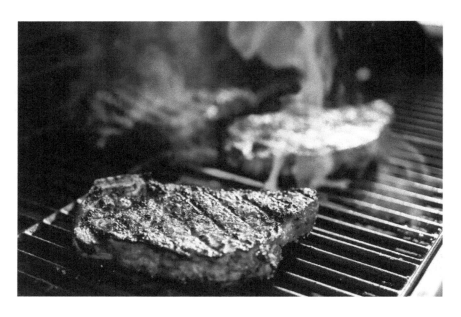

# 1. Chicken Meatballs

**Preparation Time:** 30 minutes
**Cooking Time:** 25 minutes
**Servings:** 2
**Total budget**: 10$
**Ingredients**

- 12 oz. chicken, minced
- ½ onion, chopped finely
- 3 tbsps. sage leaves, chopped
- 1 egg
- 2 ½ oz. breadcrumbs
- 1 lemon, grated zest
- 3 ribs celery
- 2 tbsps. canola oil
- Sea salt
- White pepper
- 4 oz. white wine
- 4 oz. chicken stock
- 4 oz. parmesan, grated
- 8 oz. cream
- Arugula

**Directions**

Mix the minced chicken, onion, egg, sage, celery, salt, lemon zest, breadcrumbs, pepper, and salt in one bowl. Divide the mixture into 12 portions. Pick up each portion and roll it in your palm. In this way, make 12 balls with the mixture and put them in one baking tray that has been lined. Keep it in the refrigerator for ten min. Heat some oil in one pan on the stovetop and fry the meatballs until they become golden brown. It takes about 10 to 15 min. Remove the meatballs and place them on one paper towel to get rid of the excess oil. In the meantime, put the chicken stock, cream, and wine in a pan. Simmer the sauce until it becomes thick and is reduced in quantity. Put the meatballs in the pan and cook for a few minutes. Garnish with grated parmesan and arugula. Serve it with rice or slices of bread.

**Nutrition**
**Calories:** 549 kcal   **Total Fat:** 30.6 g   **Protein:** 39.8 g

## 2. Caprese Turkey Burgers

**Preparation Time:** 10 minutes
**Cooking Time:** 10 minutes
**Servings:** 2
**Total budget**: 10$

## Ingredients

- ½ lb. 93% lean ground turkey
- 2 (1,5-oz.) whole wheat hamburger buns, toasted
- ¼ cup mozzarella cheese, shredded
- 1 egg
- 1 big tomato
- 1 small clove garlic
- 4 large basil leaves
- ⅛ tsp. salt
- ⅛ tsp. pepper

## Directions

Combine turkey, white egg, minced garlic, salt, and pepper, mix until combined. Shape into 2 cutlets. Put cutlets into a skillet; cook 5 to 7 min per side. Top cutlets properly with cheese and sliced tomato at the end of cooking. Put 1 cutlet on the bottom of each bun. Top each patty with 2 basil leaves.

## Nutrition

**Calories:** 180 kcal    **Total Fat:** 4 g    **Protein:** 7 g

## 3. Chicken and Chickpeas

**Preparation Time:** 15 minutes
**Cooking Time:** 15 minutes
**Servings:** 2
**Total budget**: 9$

### Ingredients

- 1 lb. chicken thighs, boneless, and skinless
- 1 (5-oz.) pkg baby spinach
- 1 cup chicken broth
- 1½ tsp. garlic
- 1 (15-oz.) can chickpeas
- 1½ tsp. seasoning blend
- ½ (6-oz.) can tomato paste
- 1 tbsp. olive oil
- ½ tsp. salt
- ¼ tsp. pepper

### Directions

Sprinkle chicken with salt and pepper. Cook 4 minutes per side until browned. Remove. Add minced garlic to skillet; cook until fragrant. Add tomato paste; cook 2 minutes. Add drained and rinsed chickpeas, broth, and seasoning; cook 5 minutes. Stir spinach into chickpea mixture. Cook 2 minutes and return chicken to skillet and cook 1 to 2 minutes.

### Nutrition

**Calories:** 170 kcal    **Total Fat:** 7 g    **Protein:** 25 g

# Lunch Fish and Seafood Recipes

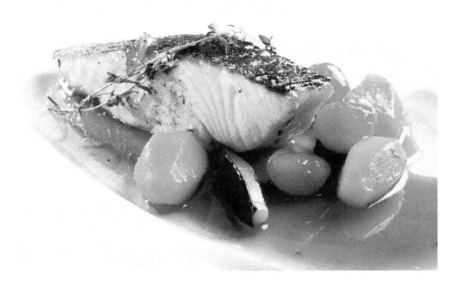

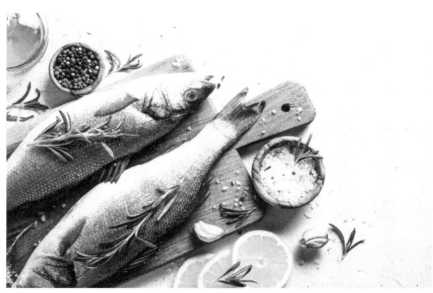

**1. Salmon and Brussels Sprouts**
**Preparation Time:** 15 min
**Cooking Time:** 25 min
**Servings:** 2
**Total budget**: 15$
**Ingredients**

- 3 (6-oz.) salmon fillets
- ⅓ cup chicken broth
- 5 large cloves garlic
- 1 lb. Brussel sprouts
- 2 tbsps. olive oil
- 1 tbsp. flat-leaf parsley, fresh
- ½ tsp. salt, divided
- ¼ tsp. pepper, divided

**Directions**

Preheat oven to 450°F. Mince 1 clove garlic; add oil, ¼ tsp. finely chopped parsley, ¼ tsp. salt, and ⅛ tsp. pepper. Cut trimmed Brussel sprouts in half. Cut 4 cloves garlic in half; mix with Brussel sprouts and 1½ tbsp. oil mixture. Bake 15 minutes. Remove from oven. Arrange salmon on top of Brussel sprouts. Combine broth and remaining oil mixture, drizzle over salmon. Sprinkle with 1½ tsp. parsley, ¼ tsp. salt, and ⅛ tsp. pepper. Bake 10 to 15 minutes.

**Nutrition**
**Calories:** 210 kcal    **Total Fat:** 19 g    **Protein:** 20 g

**2. Seafood Paella**
**Preparation Time:** 10 mins
**Cooking Time:** 10 mins
**Serving:** 2
**Total budget**: 15$
**Ingredients**
**Fish stock:**

- 6 cups water
- 1 bunch parsley
- 1 bay leaf
- 1 stalk celery
- 2 carrots
- 4 fish head

**Paella:**

- 1 cup shirataki rice
- 1 cup shellfish, mixed
- 5 cups seafood
- 1 pinch turmeric
- 1 cup low-sodium vegetable stock
- 5 green bell pepper, diced
- 5 red bell pepper
- 2 tsps. ghee
- 5 onion, diced

## Directions

To make the fish stock, add the ingredients to the Instant Pot cooker before sealing it and selecting the high pressure setting for 5 minutes. All the pressure to naturally release when the timer goes off. Set the stock aside. To make the paella, start by setting the Instant Pot to sauté before adding in the ghee and allowing it to heat up fully before adding in the onion and peppers and allowing them to cook for about 3 minutes or until the onion begins to brown and soften. Add in the rice and the seafood and let everything cook approximately 2 min. Reintroduce the fish stock along with the turmeric and mix well. Place shellfish on top (if applicable) but do not mix. Seal the lid of the cooker, choose the high pressure, and set the time for 6 min. Once the timer goes off, select the natural pressure release option and remove the lid as soon as the pressure has normalized. Mix well prior to serving.

## Nutrition

**Calories:** 453 kcal    **Total Fat:** 28 g   **Protein:** 30 g

**3. Instant Pot Cod**
**Preparation Time:** 10 mins
**Cooking Time:** 5 mins
**Servings:** 2
**Total budget**: 13$
**Ingredients**

- 1 tbsp. earth balance butter
- Pepper, as desired
- 8 tbsps. cherry tomatoes
- 2,6 oz. Cod filets
- 1 tbsp. olive oil

## Directions

Place a small, oven safe glass dish into your Instant Pot before placing your tomatoes inside of it. Place the cod on top of the tomatoes in a single layer before seasoning as desired and drizzling with olive oil. Seal the lid of the cooker, choose the high-pressure option and set the time for 5 min.

Once the timer goes off, select the instant pressure release option and remove the lid as soon as the pressure has normalized.

**Nutrition**
**Calories:** 263 kcal  **Total Fat:** 23.4 g  **Protein:** 18 g

# 4. Spicy Lemon Salmon

**Preparation Time:** 5 minutes
**Cooking Time:** 5 minutes
**Serving:** 2
**Total budget**: 15$

## Ingredients

- 1 cup water
- Pepper, as desired
- 1 tbsp. Nanami Togarashi
- 1 Lemon, juiced, 1 sliced
- 2 Salmon filets (2, 6 oz.)

## Directions

Season the salmon using the pepper, Nanami, and lemon juice. Place trivet in the bottom of the Instant Pot, taking care to ensure the handles remain up. Add cup of water to the Instant Pot cooker before placing the fish on the rack and topping with any remaining juice or seasoning. Seal the lid of the cooker, choose the high-pressure option, and set the time for 5 min. Once the timer goes off, select the instant pressure release option and remove the lid as soon as the pressure has normalized to prevent the fish from over cooking.

## Nutrition

**Calories:** 250 kcal   **Total Fats:** 15.4 g   **Protein:** 17 g

# Dinner Vegetable Recipes

**1. Spicy Chili Balls**

**Preparation Time:** 10 minutes

**Cooking Time:** 15 minutes

**Servings:** 2

**Total budget**: 10$

**Ingredients**

- 5 cups vegetables
- red chili
- fish stock
- 1 tsp. red pepper flakes, crushed
- 20 oz. tomatoes, preserved and sliced
- 1 cup carrots, minced into branches
- 1 green bell pepper, lightly cut
- 3 garlic cloves, cut
- 1 cup red onion, chopped
- ½ tsp. cilantro films, to embellish
- black pepper, to savor
- 2-½ cups pinto-beans, dehydrated and soaked
- 1 vessel parsnip, minced

**Directions**

Combine oil within the immediate pot cooker and arranged the container on heating mode.

Supplement onion and cook for 3–4 mins. Combine chili and bake for more extra minutes. Add stock and mix thoroughly. Put the cooking rack above the red bean batter and set squash on the shelf. Perform the slurry by speeding a flaxseed dish, including a few tbsp. boiling liquid. Replace the Slurry with the Instant Cooker Pot and beat to mix. Combine champagne or vinegar and heat for few more minutes more. Serve containers, including Garlic-croutons. Season with black pepper, flavorings, and spice, salt. Lock pot with top and bake on raised for 8-10 mins. Discharge pressure using the quick removal method, then loosen the cover. Get spoon squash inside a container. Supplement black bean ingredients and mix thoroughly. Moisten with cheese and butternuts.

**Nutrition**
**Calories:** 136 kcal    **Total Fat:** 8 g    **Carbs:** 20 g

## 2. Potato Casserole
**Preparation Time:** 10 minutes
**Cooking Time:** 15 minutes
**Servings:** 2
**Total budget**: 6$
**Ingredients**
- 5–6 large potatoes
- ¼ cup sour cream
- ½ cup butter
- 5–6 bacon strips
- 1–2 cups mozzarella cheese
- ¼ cup heavy cream

**Directions**
Place the potatoes in a pot with boiling water, cook until tender. Place the potatoes in a bowl, add sour cream, butter, cheese, and mix well. In a baking dish, place the bacon strips and cover with potato mixture. Add remaining mozzarella cheese on top. Bake at 325°F for 15–18 mins or until the mozzarella is fully melted. If ready, remove all of it from the oven and serve.

**Nutrition**
**Calories:** 276 kcal   **Total Fat:** 6.9 g   **Protein:** 21.9 g

### 3. Potato Soup

**Preparation Time:** 10 minutes
**Cooking Time:** 50 minutes
**Servings:** 2
**Total budget**: 6$

### Ingredients

- 1 onion
- 2–3 carrots
- 2 tbsps. flour
- 5–6 large potatoes
- 2 cups milk
- 2 cups bouillon
- 1 cup water
- 2 cups milk
- 1 tsp. salt
- 1 tsp. pepper

### Directions

In a saucepan, melt butter and sauce carrots, garlic, and onion for 4–5 mins. Add flour, milk, potatoes, bouillon and cook for another 15–20 mins. Add pepper and remaining ingredients and cook on low heat for 20–30 mins. When ready, remove from heat and serve.

### Nutrition

**Calories:** 300 kcal    **Total Fat:** 9 g    **Protein:** 31 g

## 4. Butternut Squash Pizza

**Preparation Time:** 10 minutes
**Cooking Time:** 15 minutes
**Servings:** 2
**Total budget**: 8$

### Ingredients

- 2 cups butternut squash
- ¼ tsp. salt
- 1 pizza crust
- 5-6 tbsps. Alfredo sauce
- 1 tsp. olive oil
- 4–5 cups baby spinach
- 2-3 oz. goat cheese

### Directions

Place the pizza crust on a baking dish and spread the Alfredo sauce. In a skillet, sauté spinach and place it over the pizza crust. Add goat cheese, butternut squash, olive oil, and salt. Bake pizza at 425°F for 8–10 mins. If ready, remove from the oven and serve.

### Nutrition

**Calories:** 300 kcal    **Total Fat:** 9 g    **Protein:** 31 g

### 5. Tomato Wrap

**Preparation Time:** 5 minutes
**Cooking Time:** 15 minutes
**Servings:** 2
**Total budget**: 6$
**Ingredients**

- 1 cup corn
- 1 cup tomatoes
- 1 cup pickles
- 1 tbsp. olive oil
- 1 tbsp. mayonnaise
- 6–7 turkey slices
- 2–3 whole-wheat tortillas
- 1 cup romaine lettuce

**Directions**

In a bowl, combine tomatoes, pickles, olive oil, corn, and set aside. Place the turkey slices over the tortillas and top with tomato mixture and mayonnaise. Roll and serve.

**Nutrition**

**Calories:** 300 kcal   **Total Fat:** 9 g   **Protein:** 31 g

## 6. Veggie Stir-Fry

**Preparation Time:** 5 minutes
**Cooking Time:** 15 minutes
**Servings:** 2
**Total budget**: 7$

### Ingredients

- 1 tbsp. cornstarch
- 1 garlic clove
- ¼ cup olive oil
- ¼ head broccoli
- ¼ cup show peas
- ½ cup carrots
- ¼ cup green beans
- 1 tbsp. soy sauce
- ½ cup onion

### Directions

In a bowl, combine garlic, olive oil, cornstarch and mix well. Add all the ingredients and toss to coat. In a skillet, cook vegetables mixture until tender. When ready, transfer to a plate, garnish with ginger, and serve.

### Nutrition

**Calories:** 200 kcal     **Total Fat:** 9 g     **Protein:** 20 g

# Dinner Meat Recipes

**1. Chicken Alfredo**

**Preparation Time:** 10 minutes

**Cooking Time:** 10 minutes

**Servings:** 2

**Total budget**: 11$

**Ingredients**

- 2–3 chicken breasts
- 1 lb. rotini
- 1 cup parmesan cheese
- 1 cup olive oil
- 1 tsp. salt
- 1 tsp. black pepper
- 1 tsp. parsley

**Directions**

In a pot, add the rotini and cook on low heat for 12–15 mins. In a frying pan, heat olive oil, add chicken, salt, parsley, and cook until the chicken is brown. Drain the rotini and place the rotini in the pan with chicken.Cook for 2–3 mins. When ready, remove from heat and serve with parmesan cheese on top.

**Nutrition**

**Calories:** 286 kcal    **Total Fat:** 11 g    **Protein:** 30 g

## 2. Chicken Salad with Ginger and Sesame Dressing

**Preparation Time:** 30 minutes
**Cooking Time:** 25 minutes
**Servings:** 2
**Total budget**: 10$
**Ingredients**

- 3 oz. chicken breast, shredded, cooked
- 4 cups romaine lettuce, chopped
- 4 oz. spinach, fresh
- 2 oz. carrot, shredded
- 10 oz. radish, sliced
- 1 scallion, cut into slices
- 3 tbsps. ginger-sesame dressing, prepared

**Directions**

Combine the chicken, lettuce, spinach, radishes, scallion, and carrots into one bowl. Add the prepared ginger-sesame dressing. Toss the contents, so it mixes well with the dressing. You can serve it with rice or noodles.

**Nutrition**

**Calories:** 71 kcal   **Total Fat:** 1.1 g   **Protein:** 6.6 g

**3. Mortadella & Bacon Balls**
**Preparation Time:** 10 minutes
**Cooking Time:** 30 minutes
**Total budget**: 9$
**Servings:** 2
**Ingredients**

- 4 oz. Mortadella sausage
- 4 bacon slices, cooked and crumbled
- 2 tbsps. almonds, chopped
- ½ tsp. Dijon mustard
- 3 oz. cream cheese

## Directions
Combine the mortadella and almonds in the bowl of your food processor. Pulse until smooth.Whisk the cream cheese and mustard in another bowl. Make balls out of the mortadella mixture.

Make a thin cream cheese layer over. Coat with bacon, arrange on a plate, and chill before serving.

**Nutrition**
**Calories:** 547 kcal    **Total Fat:** 51 g    **Protein:** 21.5 g

## 4. Noodle Soup

**Preparation Time:** 10 minutes
**Cooking Time:** 15 minutes
**Servings:** 2
**Total budget**: 6$
**Ingredients**

- 2–3 cups water
- 1 can chicken broth
- 1 tbsp. olive oil
- ¼ red onion
- ¼ cup celery
- ¼ tsp. salt
- ¼ tsp. black pepper
- 5–6 oz. fusilli pasta
- 2 cups chicken breast
- 2 tbsps. Parsley

**Directions**

In a pot, boil water with broth. In a saucepan, heat oil, add carrot, pepper, celery, onion, salt and sauté until tender. Add broth mixture to the mixture and pasta. Cook until al dente and stir in chicken breast, cook until chicken breast is tender. When ready, remove from heat, stir in parsley, and serve.

**Nutrition**

**Calories:** 784 kcal    **Total Fat:** 39.8 g    **Carbs:** 23.8 g
**Protein:** 78.3 g    **Fiber** 4.4 g

## 5. Penne with Asparagus
**Preparation Time:** 10 minutes
**Cooking Time:** 20 minutes
**Servings:** 2
**Total budget**: 9$
### Ingredients
- 6-7 oz. penne pasta
- 2-3 bacon slices
- ¼ cup red onion
- 2 cups asparagus
- 1 cup chicken broth
- 2-3 cups spinach leaves
- ¼ cup parmesan cheese

### Directions
Cook pasta until "al dente". In the skillet, cook the bacon until it is crispy and set aside. In a pan add onion, asparagus, broth and cook on low heat for 5-10 mins. Add spinach, cheese, pepper, pasta and cook for another 5-6 mins. When ready, sprinkle bacon and serve.

### Nutrition
**Calories:** 286 kcal      **Total Fat:** 15 g      **Protein:** 35 g

# Dinner Fish and Seafood

**1. Cheese Stuffed Shells**
**Preparation Time:** 20 minutes
**Cooking Time** 25 minutes
**Servings:** 2
**Total budget**: 10$
**Ingredients**

- 2-3 cups macaroni
- 2 cups cream cheese
- 1 cup spaghetti sauce
- 1 cup onions
- 1 cup mozzarella cheese

**Directions**

In a pot boil water and add shells. Cook for 12–15 mins. In a baking dish add spaghetti sauce. In a bowl combine cream cheese, onion and set aside. Add cream cheese to the shells and place them into the baking dish. Bake at 325°F for 30 mins or until golden brown. When ready, remove the oven and serve.

**Nutrition**
**Calories:** 363 kcal    **Total Fat:** 72.5 g    **Carbs:** 124.1 g
**Protein:** 54.5 g

**2. Thyme Cod**
**Preparation Time:** 5 minutes
**Cooking Time:** 15 minutes
**Servings:** 2
**Total budget**: 10$
**Ingredients**
- 1 tbsp. olive oil
- ½ red onion
- 1 can tomatoes
- 2-3 springs thyme
- 2-3 cod fillets

**Directions**
In a frying pan, heat the olive oil and sauté onion, stir in tomatoes, spring thyme, and cook for 5–6 mins. Add cod fillets, cover, and cook for 5–6 mins per side. When ready, remove from heat and serve.

**Nutrition**
**Calories:** 186 kcal    **Total Fat:** 7.6 g    **Carbs:** 5.8 g
**Protein:** 23.1 g

### 3. Tuna Salad

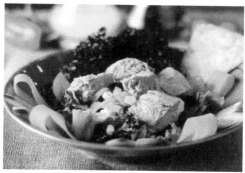

**Preparation Time:** 15 minutes
**Cooking Time:** 15 minutes
**Servings:** 2
**Total budget**: 10$
## Ingredients
- 2 (5 oz.) cans water tuna, packed and drained
- 2 tbsps. plain Greek yogurt, fat-free
- Salt and ground black pepper, as required
- 2 medium carrots, peeled and shredded
- 2 apples, cored and chopped
- 2 cups spinach, fresh and torn

## Directions
In a large bowl, add the tuna, yogurt, salt, and black pepper and gently, stir to combine. Add the carrots and apples and stir to combine. Serve it immediately.

## Nutrition
**Calories:** 306 kcal   **Total Fat:** 1.8 g   **Protein:** 35.8 g

# Appetizers and Side Dishes

## 1. Balsamic Green Beans with Bacon and Pine Nuts

**Preparation Time:** 18-20 minutes
**Cooking time:** 25 minutes
**Servings:** 2
**Total budget**: 10$

**Ingredients**

- 2 slices bacon
- 1 lb. green beans, frozen, french slice
- ¼ medium onion
- 1 tbsp. olive oil
- 1 tbsp. butter
- 1 tbsp. marjoram, dried
- ¼ cup (35g) pine nuts, toasted
- 2 tbsps. (28 ml) balsamic vinegar

## Directions

First, lay your bacon on a microwave bacon rack or in a glass pie plate. Nuke it for 2 minutes on high, or until crisp. Remove from the microwave, drain, and reserve. While the bacon's cooking, put your green beans, still frozen, in a microwavable casserole dish with a lid. Add a couple of tbsps. (30 ml) water, cover, and when the bacon is done, put them in the microwave for 7 mins on high.

Slice up your onion; you want it finely minced. Now coat your big skillet with nonstick cooking spray, put it over medium heat, and add the olive oil and butter. When the butter's melted, swirl it into the olive oil, then add the onion. Sauté for just a few minutes, till the onion is translucent. Stir in the marjoram. Turn off the heat if the beans are not done yet - it is better than burning your onion! When the microwave beeps, stir your green beans, and give them 3 more minutes. You want them tender, but not overcooked. **Note:** If your pine nuts are not toasted, you will require to do that, too. Spread them in a shallow pan and give them 7 or 8 minutes at 325°F. A toaster oven is perfect for this, who wants to heat up the oven for a little job like this? But many stores carry pre toasted pine nuts.

**Nutrition**

**Calories:** 73 kcal   **Total Fat:** 5 g   **Protein:** 3 g

**2. Sweet-And-Sour Cabbage**
**Preparation Time:** 18-20 minutes
**Cooking Time:** 25 minutes
**Servings:** 2
**Total budget**: 9$
**Ingredients**

- 3 slices bacon
- 4 cups cabbage, shredded
- 2 tbsps. cider vinegar
- 12 drops liquid stevia, English toffee

**Directions**

In a heavy skillet, cook the bacon until crisp. Remove and drain. Add the cabbage to the bacon grease and sauté it until tender-crisp about 10 mins. Stir together the vinegar and stevia. Stir this into the cabbage. Crumble in the bacon just before serving, so it stays crisp.

**Nutrition**
**Calories:** 46 kcal   **Total Fat:** 3 g   **Protein:** 2 g

### 3. Dragon's Teeth

**Preparation Time:** 18–20 minutes
**Cooking Time:** 25 minutes
**Servings:** 2
**Total budget**: 10$

### Ingredients

- 1 head Napa cabbage
- ¼ cup (60g) chili garlic paste
- 2 tbsps. (28 ml) soy sauce
- 2 tbsps. dark sesame oil
- 1 tbsp. salt
- 12 drops liquid stevia, plain
- 2 tbsps. (28 ml) peanut or canola oil
- 2 tbsps. rice vinegar

### Directions

I like to slice my head Napa cabbage in half lengthwise, then lay it flat-side down on the soliciting board and slice it about ½-inch (1 cm) thick. Slice it one more time, lengthwise down the middle, and then do the other half head. Mix the chili garlic paste, soy sauce, sesame oil, salt, and stevia in a small dish, and set by the stove. In a wok or extra-large skillet, over the highest heat, heat the peanut or canola oil. Add the cabbage and start stir-frying. After about a minute, add the seasoning mixture and keep stir-frying until the cabbage is just starting to wilt, you want it still crispy in most places. Sprinkle in the rice vinegar, stir once more, and serve.

### Nutrition

**Calories:** 175 kcal **Total Fat:** 9 g

## 4. Roasted Asparagus

**Preparation Time:** 25 minutes
**Cooking Time:** 7–12 minutes
**Servings:** 10
**Total budget**: 10$
**Ingredients**

- 3 lbs. (1.4 kg) asparagus,
- 1 tbsp. (15 ml) olive oil
- Salt and ground black pepper, to taste

### Directions

Preheat oven to 450°F (230°C). Gently bend each asparagus stalk until it snaps, or breaks. Toss the part that was below the break. Pour the olive oil into an ovenproof dish or shallow baking pan large enough to accommodate the asparagus. Add salt and pepper, freshly ground is best, to taste. Place the asparagus in the olive oil and roll it in the oil and seasonings until it is well coated. Place in the preheated oven and roast until just tender, 5 to 7 mins for thin spears, 8 to 10 for medium, 10 to 12 for thick. Remove and serve immediately. You can easily top the asparagus with favorite sauces or melt butter until golden brown and pour over the top, but it is delicious just as is! Adjust the amount of oil and seasonings for larger or smaller quantities of asparagus.

### Nutrition

**Calories:** 19 kcal    **Total Fat:** 1 g    **Protein:** 2 g

## 5. Asparagus with Curried Walnut Butter
**Preparation Time:** 20 minutes
**Cooking Time:** 30 minutes
**Servings:** 2
**Total budget**: 8$
**Ingredients**
- 1-lb. (455g) asparagus
- ¼ cup (55g) butter
- 2 tbsps. (15g) walnuts, chopped
- 1 tbsp. curry powder
- ½ tbsp. ground cumin
- 9 drops liquid stevia, English toffee

**Directions**
Snap the ends off the asparagus where they want to break naturally. Put in a microwavable container with a lid, or use a glass pie plate and plastic wrap. Either way, add 1 tbsp. or 2 (15 to 28 ml) water, and cover. Microwave on high for 5 mins. Do not forget to uncover as soon as the microwave goes beep, or your asparagus will keep cooking and be limp and sad! While that is cooking, put the butter in a medium skillet over medium heat. When it is melted, add the walnuts. Stir them around for 2 to 3 mins, until they are getting toasty. Now stir in the curry powder, cumin, and stevia, and stir for another 2 mins or so. Your asparagus is done by now. Fish it out of the container with tongs, put it on your serving plates, and top with the curried walnut butter.

**Nutrition**
**Calories:** 189 kcal    **Total Fat:** 19 g    **Protein:** 3 g

## 6. Cauliflower Recipe
**Preparation Time:** 20 minutes
**Cooking Time:** 20 minutes
**Servings:** 2
**Total budget**: 6$
## Ingredients
- 4 slices bacon
- ½ head cauliflower + ½ green bell pepper
- ½ medium onion
- ¼ cup (25 g) olives, stuffed and sliced

## Directions
Chop the bacon into small bits and start it frying in a large, heavy skillet over medium-high heat. Chop the cauliflower into ½-inch (1 cm) bits. Chop up the stem, too; no need to waste it. Put the chopped cauliflower in a microwavable casserole dish with a lid, or a microwave steamer if you have one, add a couple of tbsps. (28 ml) water, cover, and microwave for 8 minutes on High. Give the bacon a stir, then go back to the chopping board. Dice the pepper and onion. By now, some fat has cooked out of the bacon, and it is starting to brown around the edges. Add the pepper and onion to the skillet. Sauté until the onion is translucent and the pepper is beginning to get soft. By then, the cauliflower should be done, and then add it to the skillet without draining and stir - the extra little bit of water is going to help dissolve the bacon flavor from the bottom of the skillet and carry it through the dish. Stir in the olives, let the whole thing cook another minute while stirring.

## Nutrition
**Calories:** 49 kcal    **Total Fat:** 4 g    **Protein:** 2 g

# Snack and Dessert

## 1. Pumpkin Custard

**Preparation Time:** 30 minutes
**Cooking Time:** 2 h
**Servings:** 2
**Total budget:** 6$
**Ingredients**

- ½ cup  almond flour
- 4 eggs
- 1 cup pumpkin puree
- ½ cup  stevia/erythritol blend, granulated
- ⅛ tsp. sea salt
- 1 tsp. vanilla extract or maple flavoring
- 4 tsps. butter, ghee, or coconut oil, melted
- 1 tsp. pumpkin pie spice

## Directions

Grease or spray a slow cooker with butter or coconut oil spray. In a medium mixing bowl, beat the eggs until smooth. Then add in the sweetener. To the egg mixture, add in the pumpkin puree along with vanilla or maple extract. Then add almond flour to the mixture along with the pumpkin pie spice and salt. Add melted butter, coconut oil, or ghee.  Transfer the mixture into a slow cooker. Close the lid. Cook for 2-2 ¾ hours on low. When through, serve with whipped cream, and then sprinkle with little nutmeg if need be. Set slow cooker to the low setting. Cook for about 2-2.45 hours and begin checking at the two-hour mark. Serve warm with stevia whipped cream and a sprinkle of nutmeg.

**Nutrition**
**Calories:** 147 kcal   **Total Fat:** 12 g   **Protein:** 5 g

## 2. Blueberry Lemon Custard Cake

**Preparation Time:** 30 minutes
**Cooking Time:** 3 h
**Servings:** 2
**Total budget:** 9$
**Ingredients**

- 6 eggs, separated
- 2 cups light cream
- ½ cup coconut flour
- ½ tsp. salt
- 2 tsps. lemon zest
- ½ cup sugar substitute, granulated
- ⅓ cup lemon juice
- ½ cup blueberries fresh
- 1 tsp. lemon liquid stevia

## Directions

Into a stand mixer, add the egg whites and whip them well until stiff peaks have formed; set aside.

Whisk the yolks with the remaining ingredients except blueberries, to form batter. When done, fold egg whites into the formed batter a little at a time until slightly combined. Grease the crock pot and then pour in the mixture. Sprinkle batter with the blueberries. Close the lid and cook for 3 hours on low. When the cooking time is over, open the lid and let cool for an hour, and let chill in the refrigerator for at least 2 hours or overnight. Serve cold with little sugar-free whipped cream.

## Nutrition

**Calories:** 165 kcal    **Total Fat:** 10 g    **Carbs:** 14 g
**Protein:** 4 g

CPSIA information can be obtained
at www.ICGtesting.com
Printed in the USA
BVHW091055090621
609091BV00009B/1020

9 781802 224993